# DR. SEBI ALKALINE DIET RECIPE BOOK

A Complete Self-Guided Approach to Prepare Dr. Sebi's Alkaline Electric Recipes with Step By Step Method of Preparation

**Green Wood**

# Acknowledgment

The works of late Dr. Sebi is the foundation on which this book was made, and his immense efforts on improving human health and preventing diseases cannot go unappreciated.

My immense gratitude goes to my research partner, Mr. Oluwafemi Oyenekan, for his massive input in helping put this piece together; his indigenous knowledge of organic herbs formulation is remarkable.

# Dedication

I dedicate this book to Almighty God, who opened our eyes to the health benefits of herbal products.

# Table of Contents

vii

The forest not only hides man's enemies, but it's full of man's medicine, healing power, and food.

- You don't have to quit eating; all you need to do is eat healthily
- Nature itself is the best physician
- The plants have enough spirit to transform our limited vision
- Whenever the immune system successfully deals with an infection, it emerges from the experience stronger and better able to confront similar threats in the future. Our immune system develops in combat. If, at the first sign of infection, you always jump in with antibiotics, you do not give the immune system a chance to grow stronger. – (Andrew Weil, MD)

# Introduction

The ideology behind the concept of this book can be traced to the concept developed by a famous pathologist and herbalist who was popularly known as Dr. Sebi (Birth Name: Alfredo Bowman). The late naturalist spent years in the study of herbal plants and products across America and Africa, as well as the Caribbean.

The Honduras-born created a line of natural vegetable cell food compounds that were used for cellular revitalization and cleansing. Dr. Sebi's diet is a plant-based diet, which is also referred to as <u>Dr. Sebi's alkaline diet</u>. The diet claims to eliminate toxic waste through alkalizing the blood, thereby rejuvenating the cells.

You might have heard or learnt that Dr. Sebi's alkaline diet is not sustainable or not easy to follow; it is far from the truth. In this book, you will get handy varieties of recipes that you can make in the comfort of your home in line with Dr. Sebi's list of recommended food lists.

This book is designed to help you transit successfully from human-made acidic food into alkaline diets, which are needed to revitalize your system, detoxify the liver, reduce blood pressure, and overall body healing.

It is important to eat, but it is more important to eat healthily.

# What is Dr. Sebi Alkaline Diet all about?

## Evolution of Dr. Sebi

Dr. Sebi was a self-educated pathologist and herbalist (Original name: Alfredo Bowman), who was born in Honduras in 1933 but was of African descent. He claimed that the western medical approach wasn't effective in treating his ailments (asthma, diabetes, and impotence). Meanwhile, he visited an herbalist in Mexico who healed him. This was the beginning of his search for herbal solutions to combating several health diseases.

It was also reported that Dr. Sebi healed Michael Jackson in 2004 before his trial on charges of child abuse. He also had celebrity clients

who approached him for herbal
Healing. Some of them were
celebrities such as Eddie Murphy,
Lisa Lopes, Steven Seagal, to
mention but a few.

*Do you know?*

*Dr. Sebi was not a medical doctor;
neither did he obtain a Ph.D.*

He formulated his diet for those who
wish to prevent or cure diseases or
improve their overall health
naturally without overly relying on
western medicine.

## His Ideology about Health, Disease, and Diet

Dr. Sebi reveals that diseases are a
result of mucus build-up in a specific
area of the body. He further
explained that a build-up of mucus
in the pancreas causes diabetes; it
also means that a build-up of mucus
in the lungs is pneumonia. He

stressed that disease could not thrive in an alkaline medium but acidic medium. In other words, an alkaline body environment promotes healthy living. In contrast, an extremely acidic body environment is a perfect breeding site for diseases.

He made a massive claim that strict adherence to his formulated herbal alkaline diet can help detoxify one's diseased body and restore it to its natural alkaline state.

Dr. Sebi's diet is largely considered as a vegan diet as it does not permit animal products at all. His diet consists of a specific list of approved fruits, grains, vegetables, nuts, seeds, oil, and herbs. His diet emphasizes consuming food products and supplements that significantly cut down or removes disease-causing mucus.

## Dr. Sebi Diet vs. Vegan Diet: The Similarities and Differences

It is right to compare Dr. Sebi closely with a vegan diet, as there are slight differences between them. Dr. Sebi's diet prohibits soy products, legumes, beans, while a vegan diet allows these proteinous meals. Consequently, Dr. Sebi's diet doesn't guarantee adequate protein consumption.

A typical vegan diet allows the consumption of all kinds of fruits and vegetables. In contrast, Dr. Sebi allows certain fruits and vegetables whose end products are deemed alkaline.

# Raisin Pancakes

## Ingredients

- 2 cups of Kamut flour
- ¼ cup of raisins
- 2 teaspoons of vanilla extract
- 1½ cup of almond milk
- 1½ teaspoon of sea moss powder
- 1 cup of maple crystals

## Preparation

- Put the Kamut flour in a bowl; add the sea-moss powder in the same bowl. Add the maple crystals, raisins, and vanilla extract to the mixture.
- Stir the mixture in almond milk.
- Pour in the resulting mixture into a heated pan and cook on both sides (evenly).

# Sea moss Breakfast Shake

## Ingredients

- 1 cup of maple syrup
- 1 teaspoon of sea moss
- 3 cups of almond milk
- 3 teaspoons of vanilla extract
- 4 bp of almond butter
- 4 cups of hot water

## Preparation

- Add boiling water and sea-moss in a blender, and blend for 1 minute.
- Add almond butter, maple syrup, vanilla extract, and almond milk.
- Blend further until it becomes smooth. Serve!

# Papaya Breakfast Shake

## Ingredients

- ½ cup of fresh or frozen papaya
- 2 cups of almond milk
- 1 teaspoon of sea moss powder
- ½ cup of agave nectar
- ½ cup of cold water

## Preparation

- Put the sea moss powder in a blender, add water, and blend for a minute.
- Add the papaya, almond milk, and agave nectar.
- Blend the mixture and blend it till smooth. Serve!

# Cream of Rye

## Ingredients

- 1 teaspoon of vanilla extract
- 1½ cup of cream of rye
- ½ cup of water
- ½ cup of almond milk
- ¼ cup of agave nectar

## Preparation

- In a pot, add water and allow boiling. Take off the fire while boiling.
- Add cream of rye and mix until it thickens.
- Add vanilla extract, almond milk, and agave nectar.
- Stir and serve.

# Cream of Kamut

## Ingredients

- 1½ cup of Kamut flour
- 1½ teaspoon of vanilla extract
- 1 cup of maple crystals
- 1 teaspoon of cinnamon
- 1½ cups of water
- 4 cups of almond milk

## Preparation

- Follow the same preparation procedure for <u>Cream of Rye</u>.

# Spelt Strawberry Waffles

## Ingredients

- 2 cups of spelt flour
- 6 strawberries
- 1 teaspoon of sea moss
- 1 teaspoon of vanilla extract
- ½ cup of almond milk
- ¼ cup of agave nectar
- ¼ cup of water

## Preparation

- Cut the strawberries into small pieces.
- Put the spelt flour, strawberry pieces, and sea moss in a bowl.
- Add vanilla extract, agave nectar, almond milk, and then water. Mix the mixture.
- Pour the mixture into a waffle maker and cook.

# Wild Rice

## Ingredients

- 1 cup mushrooms (oyster or brown button; finely chopped)
- 1 medium yellow onion (finely chopped)
- 1 small red pepper
- 1 teaspoon of sea salt
- 1 teaspoon thyme
- 1/8 cup olive oil
- 1/8 teaspoon African red pepper
- 2 teaspoons oregano
- Springwater
- Wild rice

## Preparation

- Cook the rice according to the instructions given on the package.

Set the cooked rice aside and proceed to the next procedure:

- Pour olive oil in hot frying pan or skillet.
- For 2-3 minutes, sauté the mushrooms and vegetables.
- Add African red pepper, thyme, oregano, and sea salt.
- Mix with the cooked rice and simmer for 15-20 minutes.

**Rice cooking tip**:
- For best results, soak rice overnight.

# Blueberry Spelt Muffins

## Ingredients

- ¾ cup of spelt flour
- ¾ cup of Kamut flour
- 1 cup of almond milk
- 1 cup of blueberries
- 1 teaspoon of baking powder
- ½ cup of sea moss
- 1/3 cup of maple syrup
- ¼ teaspoon of sea salt

## Preparation

- You will have to preheat your oven to 400°F.
- In a muffin pan, place the baking cups.
- In a bowl, mix the flours (spelt & Kamut), salt, baking powder, sea moss, almond milk, and syrup.

- Fold in blueberries
- Pour the mixture into baking cups and bake for at least 25 minutes.

# Kamut Puff Cereal

## Ingredients

- 1 cup of hot almond milk
- 1 cups of Kamut puffs
- ¼ cup of agave nectar
- ¼ cup of chopped almonds
- ¼ cup of chopped dates
- ¼ of raisins

## Preparation

- Add the almond milk to the other ingredients and enjoy.

# Spelt French Toast

## Ingredients

- 1 cup of almond Milk
- ½ teaspoon of sea salt
- 2 slices of spelt Bread
- 2 teaspoons of maple crystals
- 2 teaspoons of quinoa flakes
- 2 teaspoons of spelt flour

## Preparation

- Dip bread till soaking
- Add olive oil to the pan and fry on both sides lightly.

# Pasta Salad

## Ingredients

- 1½ cup of sun-dried tomatoes
- ½ cup of chopped onions
- ½ cup of olive oil
- ¼ cup of almond milk
- ¼ cup of fresh lime juice
- 2 avocados (cut in small pieces)
- 2 boxes of spelt penne
- 3 tablespoons of maple syrup
- 3 dashes of cilantro
- 2 tablespoons of sea salt

## Preparation

- Cook the pasta
- Add the other ingredients to a big bowl, and toss until it is evenly distributed.

# Mushroom Patties
## Ingredients

- 2 portabella mushrooms
- 2 tablespoons of sea salt
- 1 pinch of cayenne pepper
- 1 tablespoons dill
- 2 tablespoons onion powder
- ½ cup bell peppers
- ¼ teaspoons oregano
- ¼ bunch of cilantro
- ¼ cup of spelt flour
- 2 tablespoons olive oil

## Preparation

- Using spring water, soak the mushrooms for a minute.
- Remove the mushrooms and place them in food processor along with the bell peppers.
- Add the spelt flour, cilantro, and other seasonings.

- Mix the ingredients
  thoroughly, and then form
  patties.
- Place the formed patties in a
  heated pan containing olive
  oil.
- Fry until done. (Fry on both
  sides for about 2-3 minutes
  respectively).

# Vegetable Patties

## Ingredients

- 1 bunch of broccoli (finely chopped)
- 1 bunch of kale greens (finely cut)
- 1 medium yellow onion (finely chopped)
- 1 pinch of African red pepper
- 3 tablespoon olive oil
- ½ red and green peppers (chopped)
- ¼ cup sea moss powder
- 2 chayote squash diced
- Kamut Flour
- Spring Water

## Preparation

- Heat the skillet with the olive oil.

- Add onion, bell pepper,
  African red pepper, diced
  chayote squash, and cumin.
- Sauté for 3 minutes, and add
  kale and broccoli and simmer
  for about 10 minutes.

**Phase Two:**
- Mix sea moss with
  proportionate flour and water
  to make the dough.
- Roll out and cut into 10 inches
  diameter circles.
- Place the cooked vegetables
  onto half of the circle.
- Fold the other half without
  vegetables to cover half with
  vegetables.
- Use a fork to gently press the
  edges to close.
- Place patties on a baking
  sheet and bake for 20-30
  minutes. (Slightly grease
  baking sheet).

# Hot Veggie Wrap in Spelt Tortilla

## Ingredients

- 1 cup of diced bell peppers
- ½ cup of mushrooms chopped
- 2 cups onion
- 3 cups diced tomatoes
- Spelt Tortilla

## Preparation

- For 5 minutes, stir fry all vegetables.
- Warm spelt tortilla
- Put together

# Vegetable Mushroom Soup

## Ingredients

- 1 bunch spinach, washed and steamed
- 1 clove
- 1 cup quinoa
- 1 pound oyster mushrooms (chopped)
- 1 small red pepper (chopped)
- green bell pepper (chopped)
- ½ pound Kamut spiral pasta
- ½ teaspoon of the following:
- Marjoram
- Red pepper
- Cumin
- Rosemary
- Oregano
- Thyme.
- 2 large chayote squash (peeled & chopped)
- 2 onions (finely chopped)
- 2 tablespoons olive oil
- Springwater

# Preparation

- In a hot skillet, put the olive oil.
- Sauté mushrooms, peppers, onions, for 15-20 minutes.
- Add the mushroom mixture to a pot and fill with spring water.
- Add chayote squash, marjoram, red pepper, oregano, cumin, clove, rosemary, quinoa, and thyme.
- Simmer for 40 minutes.
- Add Kamut Pasta, and simmer for another 10-15 minutes.
- Add spinach, stir!

When the spinach is tender, you can serve.

# Vegetable Stir Fry

## Ingredients

- 1 cup broccoli (finely chopped)
- 1 pkg. oyster mushrooms (sliced)
- 1 small red and green pepper (chopped)
- ½ small yellow onions (finely chopped)
- 2 zucchini (sliced)
- 3 tablespoons olive oil
- 8 cherry tomatoes (chopped)

## Preparation

- Put olive oil in a heated stainless steel wok.
- Add onions and tomatoes.
- Add your seasonings and sauté for 3-4 minutes.

- Add mushrooms and sauté another 3-4 minutes.

# Stuffed Bell Peppers

## Ingredients

- 2 slices of Kamut or spelt bread (toasted, crumbled)
- 1½ cup of quinoa
- 1 pound oyster or brown button mushroom
- 2 green bell peppers
- 3 tablespoons olive oil
- ½ red bell peppers chopped fine
- ¼ teaspoon of ground cumin
- ½ teaspoon sweet basil
- ½ teaspoon dill
- ½ teaspoon of sea salt

## Preparation

- Steam bell pepper, until they become tender.

- In a saucepan, put the quinoa grain with water covering the top. Allow cooking on low heat until the water is absorbed. (set aside)
- Sauté the mushrooms and red bell peppers in olive oil. (Season the inside of the bell peppers with some spices).
-  Mix quinoa, red peppers, and mushrooms with seasonings.
- Stuff the bell peppers with mixture and sprinkle on bread crumbs.
- Preheat your oven to 250$^{o}$F and bake for 10-15 minutes.
- Enjoy with a green leafy salad.

# Taquitos

## Ingredients

- 2 cups of chopped onion
- 2 tablespoons oregano
- 2 tablespoons tomato sauce
- 2 teaspoons chili powder
- 2 teaspoon ground thyme
- 2 teaspoons onion powder
- 3 tablespoons of sea salt
- 4 cups of chopped mushrooms
- ¼ olive oil

## Preparation

- Add olive oil to the pan
- Add onion and sauté; add mushroom and sauté for 5 minutes.
- Add seasonings; wrap the mixture in a corn shell.
- Fry until it turns crispy.

# Spaghetti Recipe

## Ingredients

- ½ cup of olive oil
- 2 cups of tomato sauce
- 4 tablespoons of sea salt
- 2 tablespoons of onion powder
- 3 tablespoons of maple syrup
- 2 tablespoons of cayenne or chili powder (seasoning)

## Preparation

- Follow the cook instructions on the Vita Spelt Pasta package. After the pasta is cooked, allow it to strain. Set aside.

- In a saucepan, add ½ cup of olive oil, when heated;

- Add 2 cups of tomato sauce.

- Add maple syrup, along with other seasonings.

- Heat sauce for 10 minutes on a medium-high heat source.

# Whole Greens

## Ingredients

- 3 tablespoons of sea salt
- 3 bunches of mustard and turnips greens
- 2 cups of chopped onions
- ¼ cup olive oil
- 1 teaspoon of cayenne or chili powder

## Preparation

- Slightly heat the pan and add your olive oil. Add onions until it turns golden brown.

- Add the greens, and cook for 20 minutes.

- Add sea salt, cayenne/chili powder to taste.

# Lasagna

## Ingredients

- Spelt lasagna pasta
- Bay leaf, crumbled
- Almond cheddar cheese
- 8 fresh tomatoes
- 2 tablespoons olive oil
- 2 pounds mushrooms
- 1 yellow onion (chopped)
- 1 red bell pepper (chopped)
- Sea salt (to taste)
- Oregano (to taste)

## Preparation

The preparation will be in three phases:

**A. Tomato sauce**
- Add olive oil to a heated skillet.

- Add onions, oregano, bell peppers, sea salt, and bay leaf. Sauté!
- Boil the tomatoes for at least 10 minutes. Place in cold water for 5 minutes. Drain and remove tomato skin.
- Blend the tomatoes.
- Add tomato sauce in a skillet with the seasonings that have been sautéed.
- Simmer for 40-45 minutes.
- Divide the sauce into two portions, 1$^{st}$ half for mushroom sauce, and the second for layering.

## B. Mushroom sauce

- Soak mushrooms in water for a minute, stain, and slice.
- Add seasoning to taste and sauté for 2 minutes, and then add ½ portion of the prepared tomato sauce set aside for layering.

C. **Pasta**
- Cook the pasta according to its cook instructions.
- When pasta is ready, layer a deep baking dish with tomato sauce.
- Place a layer of pasta on top, then followed by a layer of mushroom sauce.
- Add a layer of almond cheddar.
- Bake for 20 minutes at 350°F until cheddar is melted.

# Mushroom Salad

## Ingredients

- ¼ bunch fresh spinach, torn
- ¼ bunch red leaf lettuce, torn
- ¼ bunch romaine lettuce, torn
- ½ pound of fresh mushrooms
- ½ red bell pepper, chopped
- 1 sm. red onion, diced
- ½ cup olive oil
- ¼ cup fresh lime juice
- ½ teaspoon dill
- ½ teaspoon basil
- ½ teaspoon of sea salt

## Preparation

- Wash mushrooms thoroughly, dry, and slice.
- Add bell pepper, onion, lime juice, dill, sea salt, and basil.

- Marinade in the refrigerator for 30 minutes.
- Wash the greens thoroughly, dry and shred.
- Mix the greens with mushrooms thoroughly.

# Vegetable Salad
## Ingredients

- ½ bunch cilantro (finely chopped)
- ½ bunch romaine lettuce, torn
- ½ bunch watercress (torn)
- ½ cup olive oil
- ½ pound fresh string beans
- ½ teaspoon dill
- ¼ cup fresh lime juice
- ¼ teaspoon cumin
- Sweet basil (to taste)

## Preparation

- In a bowl, put the olive oil.
- Add cumin, basil, dill and lime juice to the olive oil.
- Marinade for an hour (60 minutes)
- Next, thoroughly mix with watercress, lettuce, and cilantro.

# Creamy Salad Dressing

## Ingredients

- ¼ teaspoon ground cumin
- ¼ teaspoon of sea salt
- ¼ teaspoon thyme
- ½ cup fresh lime juice
- ½ teaspoon sweet basil
- 1 teaspoon maple syrup
- 2 green onions
- 2 tablespoons of spring water
- 4 tablespoons almond butter

## Preparation

- Add all the ingredients in a glass bottle.
- Shake thoroughly. Serve!

# Lime and Olive Oil Dressing

## Ingredients

- ¼ cup olive oil
- ¼ fresh lime, squeezed
- ¼ teaspoon ground cumin
- ¼ teaspoon oregano
- ¼ teaspoon sweet basil
- ¼ teaspoon thyme
- 1 tablespoon maple syrup
- 1/8 cup spring water

## Preparation

- Put all ingredients in a glass bottle.
- Shake thoroughly.

# Avocado Dressing

## Ingredients

- 3 ripe avocados (peeled and seeded)
- 4 tablespoons pure olive oil
- Pinch Cayenne Pepper
- Few sprigs of cilantro
- 1 teaspoon oregano
- 1 teaspoon cumin
- ½ small red onion
- ½ tomato (peeled)
- ½ teaspoon sweet basil
- ½ teaspoon sweet basil
- ½ teaspoon thyme
- ¼ cup fresh lime juice
- ¼ teaspoon of sea salt
- 1 teaspoon chili powder (to taste)

- 2 tablespoons spring water

# Preparation

- Put the avocados in a blender

- Add the other ingredients along with the spring water.

- Lightly blend and pour the mixture over your salad.

# Cucumber Dressing

## Ingredients

- Few sprigs of cilantro (chopped)
- 4 tablespoons pure olive oil
- 3 med. Cucumbers (peeled)
- 1½ cup spring water
- 10 almonds, raw and unsalted
- ½ teaspoon thyme
- ½ teaspoon of sea salt
- ¼ teaspoon dill
- ¼ cup green onions (chopped fine)
- ¼ cup fresh lime juice

# Preparation

- Put the spring water in a blender, and then blend the almonds in the water for about 2 minutes and set liquid aside.

- Puree the cucumbers in a blender with almonds.

- To the remaining ingredients, add olive oil, and lime juice.

- Blend lightly for about 20-30 seconds.

- Pour over your salad.

# Xave Salad Dressing

## Ingredients

- 3 tablespoons maple syrup
- 3 oz. sesame tahini
- 2 fresh limes (squeezed)
- 1 teaspoon of sea salt
- 1 oz. spring water
- ½ teaspoon red pepper

## Preparation

- Add all the ingredients in a glass bottle.
- Shake well and dress your salad.

# About the Author

Green Wood (Pen name) is a seasoned writer who focuses on herbal products and their health benefits.

His journey through some parts of the west and east Africa and Asia in search of herbal products and their health benefits stresses his passion for the application of natural organic products and their health benefits.

He has constantly been in search of natural cure and prevention of various health deficiencies.

# Author's Contact

Contact the author via his email:
greenwoodherbalhealth@gmail.com

He is open to questions, inquiries, and suggestions.

# Other Book(s) by Author:

- **The Miraculous Healing Benefits of Honey Every Home Must Have**: A DIY Self-Guided Approach to Using Honey Recipes to Heal Over 30 Health Diseases and Infections + Best Tips to Choosing Original Honey

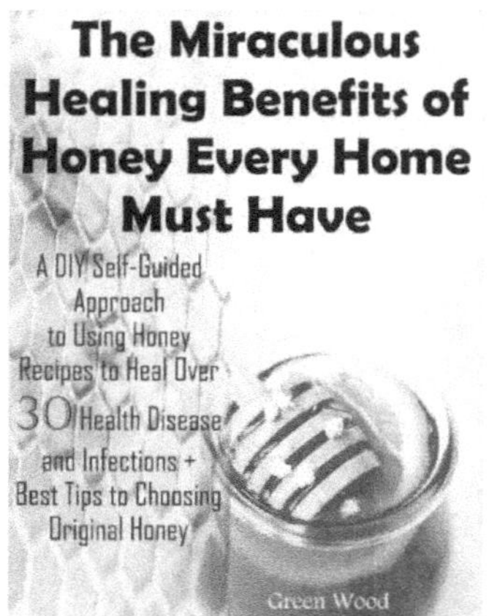


- **Dr. Sebi School of Alternative Medicine:** A Beginner's Comprehensive Guide to The Concept of Dr. Sebi Alkaline Diet+ How to Naturally Detox the Liver, Reverse Diabetes, and Mucus Cleansing

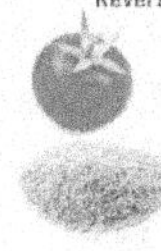
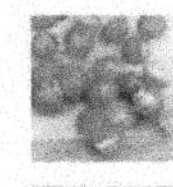
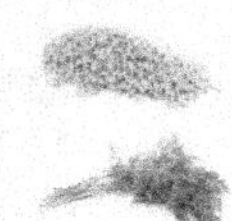
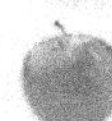


Dr. Sebi
School of Alternative Medicine
A Beginner's Comprehensive Guide to the Concept of
Dr. Sebi Alkaline Diet+ How to Naturally Detox the Liver,
Reverse Diabetes, and Mucus Cleansing
Green Wood